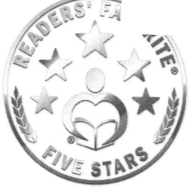

"**Choose to Lose** by Casey Hayden is dieting with the help of meals specially formulated to meet the body's needs. The help of extensive directions given to prepare the suggested menus and the ample exercises included with the plan should remove the drudgery from weight control, making it child's play. The instructions given are quite clear and concise. This, and the fact that at no stage does this book talk of dieting, always suggesting a menu instead, should endear the book to those looking for a pleasant way to shed fat."

"This is a very good book, making the tedious task of controlling one's weight a more enjoyable experience."

— ReadersFavorite.com

Choose to Lose:

A Carb Cycling Diet Plan for Rapid Weight Loss

with 50 Recipes
plus a Meal & Exercise Plan

Casey Hayden

Copyright 2015 by DiPuggo, Inc.
All rights reserved.

ISBN: 0692572023
ISBN-13: 978-0692572023

The instruction provided is offered for informational purposes solely, and is universal as so. The presentation of the information is without contract or any type of guarantee assurance.

The information is stated to be truthful and consistent, in that any liability, in terms of inattention or otherwise, by any usage or abuse of any policies, processes, or directions contained within is the solitary and utter responsibility of the recipient reader. Under no circumstances will any legal responsibility or blame be held against the publisher for any reparation, damages, or monetary loss due to the information herein, either directly or indirectly.

No part of this publication may be reproduced, duplicated, stored in a retrieval system or transmitted in any form, including electronic means, printed format, or by any other means without the prior permission in writing of the publisher, nor be circulated in writing of any publisher, nor be otherwise circulated in any form of binding or cover other than that in which it is published without a similar condition including this condition, being imposed on the subsequent purchaser. Recording of this publication is strictly prohibited without written permission from the publisher.

Respective authors own all copyrights not held by the publisher.

Any trademarks that are used are without any consent, and the publication of the trademark is without permission or backing by the trademark owner. All trademarks and brands within this book are for clarifying purposes only and are owned by the owners themselves, not affiliated with this document.

Cover photo: © Wavebreakmediamicro

Always consult with your physician or other qualified healthcare provider before embarking on a new treatment, health regimen, diet or fitness program.

DEDICATION

This book is dedicated to everyone who has ever started a
new diet or fitness program and failed. Today is a new day.
It is my goal to help you achieve your goal!

.

CONTENTS

INTRODUCTION

How many times have you started a diet only to give up a week or two later (or even sooner)? Most people trying to lose weight by dieting become very frustrated at not getting the expected results ... or any results at all. Do you end up giving in to temptation, binge-eating an entire bag of cookies, bag of chips, or a pint of Ben & Jerry's® ice cream when nobody else is in the house?

Well, you are not alone. The many thousands of people who begin diets each week, but never make it to their goal, have experienced the same aggravation. It is not an easy thing to try to lose weight. We live in a society where almost everything we consume is

1

processed, lacking in nutrients and high in calories. If you turn on the television, listen to the radio, go to a movie, or read a magazine you will be bombarded with images of carbohydrate-rich foods that are high in fat and loaded with sugar. It is no wonder we keep gaining weight! People across the globe are getting fatter and fatter at an increased rate. And to go along with our new, rounder bodies, we are less healthy. Globally, as our weight increases, so does the percentage of people with very unhealthy chronic diseases.

Diabetes, high blood pressure, coronary heart disease, sleep apnea, osteoarthritis (especially in the knees, hips and lower back), gallstones, stroke, and even cancer are all related to increased weight gain. And many people are beginning to suffer metabolic-related illnesses such as type 2 diabetes and asthma. The American Diabetes Association® estimates that 29 million Americans (or 9.3% of the population) have diabetes. 90% to 95% of those cases are Type 2 diabetes. The 2014 Global Asthma Report suggests that as many as 334 million people globally are suffering from asthma. These are very serious chronic conditions which have become an epidemic!

But trying to lose weight by strictly restricting calories, or fat intake, or carbohydrates can often lead to other problems. On your last diet, did you feel like you had no energy or had "low times" that made it hard to get anything done? Did you get acid reflux that caused your stomach and throat to burn? Did you begin to retain water and feel bloated?

For years many people have successfully minimized these kinds of complaints and achieved their weight loss goals by cycling the number of carbohydrates consumed during a specific period. This method could work for you too – if you follow the plan laid out for you in the following chapters.

Chapter One

PHASE ONE

PEOPLE WITH A healthy metabolism have systems that can take the food they eat and turn it into hormones, bone, neurotransmitters, skin, flesh, nails, and healthy organs that function at their best. This diet is about helping you to get your body to do just that. The hormones that fight depression come from food, the hormones that repair your body when it's injured come from food, the immune system that protects you from disease relies on food. You have to eat well to assist in the conversion of your food into the building blocks and fat needed for energy and health.

If you have more than ten extra pounds clinging to your frame, then your metabolism may not be working as efficiently as it ought to. If you want to get started on this diet and are serious about losing weight, then you might want to visit your doctor to get a thyroid panel, estrogen test, and testosterone test. The results of these tests can tell you a lot about your overall health and alert you to potential complications. Or, they may indicate that you're doing pretty well and just need to eat a little healthier.

The Carb Cycling Diet is about getting your body back where it needs to be in order to work *for* you rather than *against* you.

Phase one is all about your adrenal glands. Everyone has two adrenal glands that are located on top of the kidneys. They secrete stress hormones (including adrenaline and cortisol) in times of mental and physical stress. The adrenal glands will pump cortisol into your body in order to initiate the fight, flight, or freeze response.

HUMAN KIDNEYS

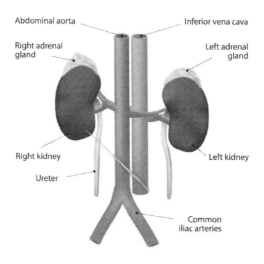

If you were really in danger, you'd run, fight, or freeze. And when the physical response was over, cortisol levels would eventually drop back to normal. However, when you're anxious and stressed over a period of time, cortisol levels remain elevated, and the body goes into a fat-storage mode. It really believes food will fix everything.

The goal of phase one is to break this cycle by telling the body that everything is all right. The adrenals need to calm down and lower the production of stress hormones, so the body knows it has everything it really needs.

There is a reason that we call certain foods "comfort foods". It's because they make us feel satiated and happy. Phase one's pasta, fruit, oatmeal, rice and toast are high-carb, low-fat foods that will naturally make you feel less stressed. These foods will have a similar effect on the adrenal glands.

Fruits such as mango, pineapple, and papaya are part of the phase one program because they're naturally higher in sugar. The sugar stimulates the pituitary gland, prompting endorphins to be released in the brain, which reduces anxiety and stress.

So what else will you be eating in phase one and what foods should you be avoiding?

Foods to Eat and Avoid

Before we get to what you're going to eat, here's the breakdown on how much food should be consumed. If you need to lose twenty pounds or less, then you'll want to stick to the following portions per meal:

• Vegetables – unlimited

- Protein – 4 oz. meat, 6 oz. fish, ½ cup cooked legumes

- Eggs – 3 whites

- Grains – 1 cup cooked or 1 oz. of crackers

- Fruit – 1 piece or 1 cup

- Fat – none added to cooking or food

- Smoothies – 1 12 oz. glass

Remember these portions are for each meal and *not* for the entire day.

If you want to lose 21-40 pounds, then multiply the above suggestions by 1 ½. If you want to lose over forty pounds, then double them. Remember, this diet is not about starvation; you should never have to feel hungry.

Safe Foods

- *Vegetables and Salad Greens:*
arrowroot, bamboo shoots, arugula, bean sprouts, beans, beet greens, beets, butternut squash, broccoli,

carrots, cabbage, chicory, celery, eggplant, cucumbers, green chilis, garlic, jicama, green onions, leeks, kale, mixed greens, lettuce, onions, mushrooms, peas, parsnips, peppers, radishes, pumpkin, spinach, rutabaga, sprouts, spirulina, tomatoes, sweet potatoes, winter squash, turnips, zucchini, yellow squash

● *Fruits:*
apples, Asian pears, apricots, berries, cherries, cantaloupe, grapefruit, figs, honeydew melon, guava, kumquats, kiwis, limes, lemons, mangos, loganberries, papaya, oranges, pears, peaches, pomegranates, pineapples, tangerines, strawberries, watermelon

● *Animal Protein:*
beef, buffalo, chicken, game, turkey, guinea fowl, deli meats, corned beef, sausage, halibut, haddock, pollock, sardines, sole, tuna, egg white

● *Vegetable Protein:*
beans, black-eyed peas, fava beans, chickpeas, lentils

● *Broth, Herbs, Spices and Condiments:*
arrowroot, baking soda, baking powder, broth, Brewer's yeast, Dijon mustard (sugar-free), cream of tartar, horseradish, dill pickles (sugar-free), mustard, ketchup (no added sugar or corn syrup), natural seasonings, liquid smoke, salsa, raw cocoa powder, tomato sauce, tamari, vanilla extract, tomato paste,

vinegar, peppermint extract, balsamic vinegar, apple cider vinegar, coconut vinegar, red wine vinegar, malt vinegar, white vinegar, fresh or dried herbs and spices

- *Sweeteners:*
Xylitol

- *Grains and Starch:*
barley, amaranth, brown rice, black barley, kamut, buckwheat, spelt, quinoa, sprouted grain, triticale, teff, wild rice, nut flours, brown rice milk, cheese and rice milk, tapioca and arrowroot flour

- *Healthy Fats:*
None

- *Beverages:*
Water, non-caffeinated herbal tea

Unsafe Foods

- Sugary foods
- Fats
- Olives and avocados
- Nuts and seeds

Importance of Exercise

Phase one is the period when you will sweat the most when it comes to exercise. Cardiovascular exercise (which raises the heart rate) is very important for the heart. In phase one, you will have a lot of extra energy from eating all those carbs, so you should easily be able to perform cardio. And along with burning off the food you just ate, you'll be burning stored fat, too!

You don't have to work out very hard to lose weight, and really, you shouldn't. Ideally, you want your heart rate to remain between 120 and 150 beats per minute. When you do cardio, try to keep the heart rate in that zone and check every now and then by taking your pulse for fifteen seconds, then multiplying by four. If you are out of breath and not able to hold a conversation, then you are working out too hard.

Try to get in thirty minutes of exercise on day one of the Carb Cycling Diet. That's it!

Sample Meal Plan

In phase one of this program, you need to eat three carb-rich, low-fat, moderate protein meals and two fruit snacks – so that's five times a day. That means you'll eat every three to four hours. Doesn't sound hard, right? And it's not!

● Breakfast could be a grain and fruit thirty minutes after you get up.

● Eat a fruit snack three hours later.

● Consume a serving of grains, protein, fruit, and a vegetable at lunch three hours later.

● Have a fruit snack three hours later.

● Consume a grain, a vegetable, and a protein at dinner three hours later.

You'll be in this phase for two days out of the week, so start on Monday and end on Tuesday.

Now that you know what your meal plan will look like, let's look at some recipes!

Chapter Two

PHASE ONE RECIPES

IN THIS CHAPTER, you'll find delicious breakfast, lunch, dinner and snack recipes for phase one of the Carb Cycling Diet.

Breakfast in Under 30 Minutes
Egg-White Soufflé
Serves: 2

Ingredients
¾ cup asparagus
¾ cup chopped red bell pepper

¼ cup chopped white onion
½ tsp. cayenne pepper
¼ tsp. sea salt
6 egg whites
1 tsp. lemon juice

Directions

1. Preheat your oven to 350 degrees F.

2. In a skillet, sauté the pepper, asparagus, and onion with a tablespoon of water until it's soft. Stir in the salt and cayenne pepper. Whip the egg whites and lemon juice with a whisk or electric mixer until stiff peaks form. Divide the egg whites into four 12 oz. ramekins. Divide the vegetables between the ramekins and fold them in gently.

3. Place the ramekins on a cookie sheet and bake twenty minutes or until the tops turn golden. Two soufflés are a portion.

Non-fat Yogurt with Fruit
Serves: 1

Ingredients

½ Cup of non-fat plain yogurt
4-5 strawberries, sliced (may substitute other fruits from safe list)
2 Tbsp. xylitol

Directions

1. Mix xylitol into the non-fat yogurt.

2. Add in strawberries and serve.

3. Keep chilled until ready to serve.

Veggie Frittata

Serves: 2

Ingredients

3 egg whites
1 egg with yolk
½ cup yellow pepper, diced
¼ cup green onion, diced
¼ cup red onion, diced
½ cup fresh button mushrooms, sliced
1 small-medium tomato, chopped
1 Tbsp. fat-free feta cheese
1 tsp. low-fat parmesan cheese (if desired)
1 sprig fresh dill, diced

Directions

1. Preheat oven to 325 degrees F.

2. Beat egg and egg whites in a bowl

3. Sauté pepper, onions and mushroom.

4. Spray a 9"x9" baking dish with a nonstick coating.

5. Pour eggs into backing dish and then add sautéed vegetables.

6. Mix in feta cheese.

7. If desired, sprinkle parmesan cheese on top of mixture.

8. Bake for 20 minutes.

Easy Lunch Recipes
Easy Oven Fajitas

Serves: 4

Ingredients

1 lb. boneless, skinless chicken breast, sliced
2 bell peppers, sliced
1 sliced onion
3 garlic cloves, minced
1 tsp. chili powder
1 tsp. cumin
½ tsp. coriander
½ tsp. paprika
¼ tsp. salt
¼ tsp. ground black pepper

Directions

1. Preheat your oven to 375 degrees F.

2. Combine the chicken, peppers, onion and garlic in a bowl.

3. In another bowl, combine the cumin, chili powder, coriander, paprika, salt and pepper.

4. Scatter the spice over the chicken and vegetables and toss to coat.

5. Bake in a 9"x11" baking dish for 20 minutes.

DIY Pizza

Serves: 2

Dough Ingredients

½ cup multi-purpose baking mix
¾ tsp. active dry yeast
2 Tbsp. plus 1 tsp. warm water
1 tsp. garlic powder
dash of pepper

Toppings Ingredients

2 ripe tomatoes, finely chopped

1/3 cup salt-reduced tomato paste

½ cup your choice of grilled chicken breast, sliced sausage, pepperoni or sardines (this allows for variety)

¼ cup your choice of green onions, peppers, spinach or broccoli

Directions

1. Preheat your oven to 375 degrees F.

2. Line a cookie sheet with parchment paper.

3. In a bowl, combine the baking mix, garlic powder, yeast and black pepper. Stir in the warm water and mix well. The mixture should look like thick soup. Set it aside for five minutes.

4. Spoon the dough into the center of some parchment paper and spread it out until it's a six-inch circle. Press the dough thin and make a ½ " ridge around the edge.

5. Pre-bake the dough for eight minutes. Remove it from the oven and add the sauce and appropriate toppings. Place it back in the oven and bake for another eight minutes.

6. Remove the pizza and slice it into four wedges. Two wedges is a serving.

Grilled Chicken & Apple Salad

Servings: 1

Ingredients

8 oz. cooked chicken breast, chopped
Uncooked spinach leaves
½ cup carrots, grated
½ cup cucumbers, sliced
½ cup cherry tomatoes
1 apple, diced
Apple Cider Vinaigrette Dressing

Directions

1. Create a bed of spinach to a plate

2. Add cucumber, carrots, tomatoes and apple.

3. Place chopped chicken breast on top vegetables.

4. Pour dressing over the entire plate as desired.

Apple Cider Vinaigrette Dressing

Serves: 2

Ingredients

6-8 Tbsp. apple cider vinegar
½ cup virgin olive oil
xylitol to taste
sea salt to taste
fresh ground pepper to taste
garlic powder to taste
splash of lemon juice (optional)
Dijon mustard to taste (optional)

Directions

1. Pour apple cider vinegar into a non-metal bowl. Gently whisk in oil.

2. Add in xylitol, salt, pepper, and garlic to taste.

3. If you prefer your dressing with some zing, then add a splash of lemon juice.

4. Add Dijon mustard as a way to add variety to your salads.

Delicious Dinner Recipes
Slow Cooker Balsamic Turkey Roast

Serves: 8

Ingredients

4 portobello mushroom caps, diced
2 cups grape tomatoes
2 cups onions, diced
¼ cup chicken broth
1/3 cup balsamic vinegar
1 Tbsp. spicy brown mustard
1 2lb. boneless turkey breast
1 tsp. dried Italian seasoning
½ tsp. garlic powder
¼ tsp. red pepper flakes
½ tsp. salt
¼ tsp. ground black pepper

Directions

1. Put the mushrooms, onions, tomatoes and broth in the bottom of a slow cooker.

2. Mix the vinegar and mustard until it's well combined. Pour it over the vegetables.

3. Rub the turkey with seasonings.

4. Place the turkey breast on top of the vegetables and cover. Cook on high for four hours or seven hours on low.

5. To serve, slice and top with the vegetables and sauce.

Jambalaya

Serves: 6

Ingredients

1 onion, chopped
1 bell pepper, chopped
2 stalks celery, diced

2 cloves garlic, minced

8 oz. skinless, boneless chicken breast, diced

3 Tbsp. Italian parsley, minced

2 bay leaves

½ tsp. cayenne pepper

28 oz. diced tomatoes

8 oz. canned tomato sauce

1 ¾ cups chicken broth

1 cup brown rice

12 oz. turkey sausage, sliced

4 oz. turkey bacon, diced

Salt

Directions

1. In a skillet or wide pot with a lid, sauté the onion, celery, bell pepper and garlic until the onion turns translucent. Add the parsley, chicken, bay leaves and cayenne pepper. Sauté for a few minutes or until the chicken is no longer pink.

2. Stir in the tomatoes, sauce, broth and rice. Bring to a boil and reduce the heat to low. Simmer for an hour or until the rice is tender.

3. Brown the sausage and bacon in a skillet over medium heat. When everything is cooked, stir ingredients together and season with salt and cayenne pepper. Serve with fresh parsley sprinkled over the

top.

Lemon Chicken with Feta

Serves: 8

Ingredients

8 boneless chicken breasts, skinned
3 Tbs. chopped green onions
3 oz. crumbled feta cheese
¼ cup lemon juice, divided
1 Tbsp. oregano leaves, divided
¼ tsp. pepper

Directions

1. Preheat oven to 350 degrees F.

2. Spray baking pan with nonstick spray.

3. Place chicken in a dish and drizzle with half of the lemon juice.

4. Sprinkle with half the oregano and all the pepper.

5. Top with cheese and onion.

6. Drizzle with remaining lemon juice and oregano.

7. Cover and bake for 45 minutes.

Green Beans with Shallots and Mushrooms
Serves: 2

Ingredients

1 lb. fresh green beans
2 shallots, sliced
1 Tbsp. tamari
12 oz. fresh mushrooms, sliced
salt and ground black pepper

Directions

1. Put the beans and a tablespoon of water in a microwave-safe bowl and cover. Microwave on high for four minutes or steam the beans for five minutes, until crisp-tender.

2. Heat a skillet over medium heat and add the tamari, shallots and a tablespoon of water. Sauté for two minutes. Add the mushrooms and sauté for another five minutes.

3. Drain the beans and stir them into the mushrooms. Season to taste and serve.

Roasted Cabbage

Serves: 4

Ingredients

½ medium green cabbage (1 ½ lbs.), outer leaves removed
1 Tbsp. extra-virgin olive oil
¼ tsp. salt
¼ tsp. freshly ground pepper

Directions

1. Preheat oven to 450 degrees F.

2. Coat a large baking sheet with nonstick cooking spray

3. Cut cabbage halves into 4 wedges.

4. Remove any think core pieces, leaving wedges as intact as possible.

5. Drizzle 1 Tbsp. olive oil onto each cut side of wedges.

6. Sprinkle ¼ tsp. salt and pepper onto each cut side of wedges.

7. Place wedges flat-side down on prepared baking sheet.

8. Roast cabbage for 12 minutes, carefully flipping over at about 8 minutes to allow each side to brown.

9. Transfer cabbage to a serving plate and drizzle with Mustard Vinaigrette while still hot.

10. May serve hot or at room temperature.

Mustard Vinaigrette

Serves: 4

Ingredients

3 Tbsp. minced fresh chives
2 Tbs. extra-virgin olive oil
2 tsp. white balsamic or white wine vinegar
2 tsp. Dijon mustard
1 tsp. lemon juice
¼ tsp. freshly ground pepper
1/8 tsp. salt

Directions

1. Combine mustard, vinegar, lemon juice, pepper, and **1/8** tsp. salt into a small bowl.

2. Add chives and olive oil

3. Stir until well combined.

Italian Dressing

Serves: 4

Ingredients

1 cup extra-virgin olive oil

¼ cup red-wine vinegar
½ onion powder
½ Tbsp. mustard powder
½ tsp granulated garlic
½ tsp Italian seasoning

Directions

1. Combine all ingredients into a dressing bottle or container that can be sealed.

2. Refrigerate until chilled.

3. When ready to use, shake vigorously until all ingredients are thoroughly mixed together.

4. Pour over fresh salad greens.

5. May also be used as a marinade for chicken. When using as a marinade, add a pinch more Italian seasoning to taste.

Snacks and Desserts
Orange Slices

Serves: 6

Ingredients

4 oranges
2 cups frozen raspberries
2 Tbsp. Xylitol
1 Tbsp. lemon juice
½ tsp. cinnamon

Directions

1. With a knife, remove the skin and pith from the oranges. Slice them crosswise and arrange them on six plates.

2. Combine the remainder of the ingredients in a saucepan and stir gently over low heat until the berries are thawed. Spoon over the oranges and serve.

Tex-Mex Black Bean Dip

Serves: 5

Ingredients

30 oz. canned black beans, rinsed
½ cup yellow onion, chopped
1/3 cup cilantro, chopped
1 garlic clove, minced
1 Jalapeno pepper, diced
2 Tbsp. lime juice
¼ tsp. cumin
¼ tsp. chili powder
½ tsp. salt
¼ tsp. ground black pepper

Directions

1. Place the beans, cilantro, onion, Jalapeno pepper, garlic, lime, cumin, salt, chili powder and black pepper in a food processor and pulse until smooth.

2. Serve with sliced vegetables. A half-cup is a serving.

Chocolate Drizzled Stuffed Strawberries
Serves: 2

Ingredients

4 large fresh strawberries, cleaned & cored
4 Tbsp. sugar-free dark chocolate
4 tsp. fat-free cream cheese
8 Tbsp. Greek yogurt
1 tsp. of real vanilla

Directions

1. Scoop out the centers of the strawberries.

2. In a bowl, combine cream cheese, Greek yogurt and vanilla.

3. In a microwave-safe bowl, melt chocolate in microwave.

4. Stuff the cheese and yogurt mixture into the strawberries

5. Drizzle the chocolate over the stuffed strawberries

6. Place in the refrigerator until chocolate is firm again

Chapter Three

PHASE TWO

PHASE TWO OF the Carb Cycling Diet is some really powerful stuff because you're actually going to be remaking and reshaping your body. The proteins and vegetables included in this phase are there for a reason. Lean proteins will provide the elements needed for your body to manufacture amino acids. And the vegetables will provide enzymes and phytonutrients to break down the proteins. These components are then converted in muscle.

Why do you want more muscle? Because muscle maintenance requires a lot of fuel and the more muscle you have, the more fat your body will burn. Having more muscle also leads to a higher metabolic rate. In phase one, you have coaxed the body to calm down and digest food rather than store fat. In phase two, food choices are designed to help you absorb protein and turn it into amino acids, releasing fat.

The exercises in phase two are focused on weight training. Using your own body weight or machines, these exercises promote small tears in the muscle, that then repairs itself, creating yet more muscle.

Foods to Eat and Foods to Avoid

Before looking at the foods you can eat and ones you can't, let's first discuss the portion sizes for this phase. [Remember to multiply by 1 ½ if you want to lose between 20 and 40 pounds and by 2 if you want to lose more weight.]

- Vegetables – unlimited
- Protein – 4 oz. meat, 6 oz. fish, or ½ cup cooked legumes
- Eggs - 3 whites
- Grains – none

- Fruit – 1 piece or 1 cup
- Fat – no additional fats
- Smoothies – 1 12 oz. glass

Remember, these portions are per meal.

Safe Foods

- *Vegetables and Salad Greens*

arugula, arrowroot, beans, asparagus, cabbage, broccoli, collard greens, celery, cucumbers, fennel, endive, garlic, scallions, kale, jicama, lettuce, leeks, mushrooms, mixed greens, onions, mustard greens, peppers, rhubarb, radishes, spinach, shallots, Swiss chard, spirulina, watercress

- *Fruits*

lemons, limes

- *Animal Protein*

beef, buffalo, game, lamb, pork, chicken, turkey, ostrich, deli meats, corned beef, jerky, turkey bacon, cod, dory, flounder, smoked salmon, halibut, sole, sardines, tuna, oysters, egg whites

- *Vegetable Protein*

None

● *Broth, Herbs, Spices and Condiments*
arrowroot, baking soda, baking powder, broth, Brewer's yeast, Dijon mustard (sugar-free), cream of tartar, horseradish, dill pickles (sugar-free), mustard, natural seasonings, liquid smoke, raw cocoa powder, tomato sauce, tamari, vanilla extract, vinegar, peppermint extract, balsamic vinegar, apple cider vinegar, coconut vinegar, red wine vinegar, malt vinegar, white vinegar
fresh or dried herbs and spices

● *Sweeteners*
Xylitol

● *Grains and Starch*
None

● *Healthy Fats*
None

● *Beverages*
Water, non-caffeinated herbal tea

Unsafe Foods

● Vegetable protein or legumes

- *Starchy Vegetables*
beets, bamboo shoots, eggplant, carrots, peas, parsnips, rutabaga, pumpkin, sweet potatoes, sprouts, winter squash turnips, potatoes, zucchini

- *Fruits*
All but lemons and limes

- Broth, Herbs, Spices and Condiments
salsa, ketchup and tomato Paste

- *Fats*
Avoid all fats, avocados, olives, nuts and seeds

Continued Exercise Routine

In phase two of the Carb Cycling diet, your body is going to get ready to build layers of muscle. Therefore, you need a weight lifting routine. If you're someone who doesn't normally lift weights, you should be lifting about ten pounds. Or, you can work with your own body weight as resistance, which is the best way to build muscle mass safely.

Pushups are a good way to promote good posture and help lift the pectorals. Try to do five in a row, take a break, and then do five more.

Another good exercise is squats. These are done as if you are sitting down in a chair, stopping before your bottom hits the seat, and standing up again. Do five squats, take a break, and then do five more.

Sample Meal Plan

When it comes to the meal plan for phase two, you're still eating five meals a day. The plan consists of three high protein, low fat, low carb meals and two protein snacks. You're still eating every three to four hours.

- *Breakfast* – have a vegetable and a protein within thirty minutes of getting up.
- *Snack* – have a protein snack three hours later.
- *Lunch* – have a vegetable and a protein lunch three hours later.
- *Snack* – another protein snack three hours later.
- *Dinner* – a protein and a vegetable dinner three to four hours later.

You'll be on this phase for two days out of the week, so choose Wednesday and Thursday to make it easy. Let's take a look at some delicious recipes for phase two of the Carb Cycling Diet!

Chapter Four

PHASE TWO RECIPES

Easy Breakfast Recipes
Fat-Blasting Baked Egg Casserole

Servings: 4

Ingredients

2 Tbsp. broth (chicken, beef or vegetable)
6 oz. cremini mushrooms, sliced

½ cup red bell pepper, chopped
2 tsp. seasoning blend
2 tsp. fresh Jalapenos, minced
2 ½ cups fresh spinach, chopped
4 oz. turkey bacon, chopped and cooked
salt and ground black pepper
9 egg whites
3 green onions, thinly sliced

Directions

1. Preheat your oven to 375 degrees F. and line a 7"x11" baking dish with parchment paper.

2. Heat a skillet and add two tablespoons of broth or water, the bell pepper, mushrooms, seasoning and Jalapenos. Cook around three minutes.

3. Add the spinach and stir until it's cooked down, around one minute. Remove it from the heat and stir in the bacon. Season with salt and pepper to taste.

4. Spread the mixture on the baking dish and whisk the egg whites. Pour them over the spinach mixture and scatter the green onions over the top.

5. Bake around twenty-five minutes. Let sit for five minutes and cut into pieces.

Homemade Breakfast Sausage

Servings: 4

Ingredients

1 lb. ground chicken
1 clove garlic, minced
1 tsp. dried sage
1 tsp. dried oregano
¾ tsp. salt
½ tsp. ground black pepper
½ tsp. red pepper flakes
 dash of nutmeg

Directions

1. Combine the ingredients in a bowl.

2. Form the patties. You should have enough for eight. Cook in a skillet until browned on both sides and cooked through.

Sweet Potato and Squash Pancakes

Servings: 6

Ingredients

2 cups shredded unpeeled sweet potato / yam
1 cup shredded unpeeled yellow squash
¼ cup shredded onion
2 egg whites or ¼ cup egg substitute
2 Tbs. chopped chives
1 Tbsp. whole wheat or brown rice flour
2 Tbsp lemon juice
1 tsp extra-virgin olive oil
½ tsp. salt
¼ tsp fresh ground pepper

Directions

1. Preheat oven to 200 degrees F.

2. Spray a griddle or 10" skillet with nonstick coconut oil spray.

3. Add olive oil to griddle or skillet

4. Heat griddle or skillet over medium heat, or to 375 degrees F.

5. Mix remaining ingredients in bowl.

6. For each pancake, spoon 1/3 cup batter onto hot griddle or skillet and flatten out the mix.

7. Cook each pancake about 5 minutes on each side or until dark brown.

8. Place cooked pancakes on ungreased cookie sheet and keep warm in the oven while the remaining pancakes are prepared.

Simple Lunch Recipes
Chicken, Red Pepper and Basil Lettuce Wrap

Servings: 2

Ingredients

8 oz. cooked chicken breast, sliced
½ cup roasted red pepper strips
½ cup red onion, sliced
2 tsp. balsamic vinegar
1 tsp. Italian seasoning
lettuce leaves
¼ cup basil, chopped

Directions

1. Stir together the first five ingredients in a bowl.

2. Spoon onto the lettuce leaves and scatter basil on top.

Salad Nicoise

Ingredients

½ lb. asparagus, trimmed
4 oz. green beans, trimmed
1 endive
1 cup lettuce leaves
6 radishes, halved
6 oz. tuna, drained
3 hard-boiled egg whites, chopped
salt and ground black pepper
lemon wedges

Directions

1. Blanch the beans and asparagus in a pot of boiling water for one minute.

2. Drain and plunge the vegetables in a bowl of ice

water.

3. Arrange the beans and asparagus on a plate along with the rest of the ingredients.

4. Season with salt and pepper and serve with a lemon wedge.

Sweet Potato Soup

Serves: 4-6

Ingredients

2 large sweet potatoes, cubed
1 onion, diced
2 carrots, diced
2 celery stalks, diced
2 cups vegetable or chicken stock
3 tablespoons olive oil
¼ tsp. ground cinnamon
dash of cayenne pepper
salt & pepper to taste

Directions

1. Preheat oven to 425 degrees F.

2. Toss the sweet potatoes in 2 tsp. olive oil, salt, and pepper.

3. Spread sweet potatoes evenly on a baking sheet covered in non-stick foil.

4. Roast sweet potatoes for 20-25 minutes until tender.

5. In a pan, sauté onions, carrots and celery in 1 Tbsp. olive oil with salt and pepper.

6. Add vegetable stock, cayenne pepper and cinnamon to the same pan.

7. Simmer for 5 minutes.

8. Purée all ingredients together in a blender.

9. Serve warm.

10. Leftovers can be frozen and served another day.

Quick Dinner Recipes
Lettuce Wraps with Smoked Salmon

Servings: 2

Ingredients

1 cucumber
1/3 cup shallots, sliced
2 Jalapeno peppers, sliced
2 Tbsp. lime juice
1 Tbsp. tamari
12 oz. smoked salmon fillets
romaine lettuce leaves
2/3 cup mint leaves
2/3 cup basil leaves

Directions

1. Use a peeler to shave the cucumber into thin ribbons. Place the ribbons in a bowl with the Jalapenos, shallots, tamari and lime juice. Allow them to marinate for 20 minutes.

2. Add the salmon and toss to blend. Scoop onto the lettuce leaves and top with mint and basil.

Quick Baked Fish with Lemons

Servings: 4

Ingredients

1 ½ lbs. cod fillets
4 lemons, sliced thinly
4 shallots, sliced thinly
¼ cup dill, minced
salt and ground black pepper

Directions

1. Preheat oven to 450 degrees F.

2. Scatter half the lemon on the bottom of a glass baking dish and sprinkle the fish with dill, salt and pepper. Lay the fish on top of the lemons.

3. Cover the fish with remaining lemon and shallot slices.

4. Bake 20 minutes uncovered. Remove the fish, lemons and shallots to a serving platter and drizzle with the pan juices.

Glazed Pork Tenderloin with Horseradish Sauce

Servings: 4

Ingredients

1 lbs. pork tenderloin
½ cup pineapple preserves
¼ tsp. salt
¼ tsp. black pepper
2 sprigs fresh rosemary
1 Tbsp. prepared horseradish

Directions

1. Preheat oven to 425 degrees F.

2. Coat a 13"x19" baking pan with coconut oil spray.

3. Combine salt and pepper, rub over pork.

4. Place one sprig of rosemary in the center of the pan.

5. Place the pork unto the pan on top of the rosemary.

6. Place the other spring of rosemary on top of the pork.

7. Bake, uncovered, for 10 minutes.

8. While the pork is baking, in a sauce pan, heat the preserves and horseradish until preserves are melted; stir until blended.

9. Remove pork from the oven.

10. Remove the top rosemary sprig from the pork.

11. Brush the pork with ¼ cup pineapple sauce.

12. Bake 10-20 minutes longer, or until thermometer put inside the pork reads 145 degrees F.

13. Remove from oven and let stand for 5 minutes before slicing.

14. Serve with remaining pineapple sauce.

Sautéed Leeks

Servings: 2

Ingredients

4 leeks, sliced
4 garlic cloves, minced
¼ cup chicken stock
lemon juice
salt and ground black pepper to taste

Directions

1. In a skillet, sauté the leeks and garlic in broth and stir until soft, around seven minutes.

2. Add the juice, salt and pepper.

Creamy Broccoli & Carrots Stir-fry

Servings: 4

Ingredients

1 ½ cups broccoli florets
1 cup carrots, thinly sliced
1 small onion, sliced and separated into rings
1 cup mushrooms, sliced
1 8 oz. can sliced water chestnuts, drained

¾ cup chicken or vegetable broth
2 tsp. ginger
1 clove garlic, chopped
¼ tsp. salt
1 Tbsp. cornstarch (or arrowroot)
2 Tbsp. oyster sauce
1 Tbsp. cold water

Directions

1. Spray skillet or wok with nonstick cooking spray and heat until it's hot.

2. Add ginger and garlic, frying for about 102 minutes until light brown.

3. Add broccoli, carrots and onion and stir for another 1-2 minutes.

4. Stir in broth and salt.

5. Cover and cook for 3 minutes or until carrots are crisp, but tender.

6. Mix cornstarch (arrowroot) and water.

7. Slowly stir liquid into vegetable mixture, stirring until thickened.

8. Add water chestnuts, mushroom and oyster sauce.

9. Continue stirring mixture as it cooks for less than 1 minute.

Cauliflower Fried Rice

Servings: 2

Ingredients

½ head cauliflower, grated (about 1 ½ cups)
2 baby carrots, shredded
2 eggs, scrambled
½ cup peas
¼ cup coconut oil
Light soy sauce to taste

Directions

1. Heat the oil in a wok or large frying pan.

2. Sauté cauliflower in oil until browned.

3. Add baby carrots and peas.

4. Push mixture to one side of the wok or pan.

5. Scramble the eggs on clear side of wok or pan.

6. When eggs are cooked, combine with cauliflower mixture.

7. Add light soy sauce to taste.

8. If desired, you can add diced chicken, pork, or shrimp into the vegetables.

Snacks and Desserts
Power Protein Dip

Servings: 2

Ingredients

3 hard-boiled egg whites
1 clove garlic
2 Tbsp. lemon juice
2 Tbsp. water
1 Tbsp. dill, minced

2 tsp. onion powder
1 tsp. sugar-free Dijon mustard
¼ tsp. salt
dash of pepper
dash of Xylitol

Directions

1. Process all ingredients in a food processor until smooth and serve with vegetables.

2. Serve with sliced vegetables. A half-cup is a serving.

Lemon Meringue Puffs

Servings: 6

Ingredients

2 large eggs whites
1 tsp fresh lemon juice
½ cup xylitol

Directions

1. Preheat over to 225 degrees F.

2. Line two baking sheets with parchment paper.

3. Prepare a pastry bag with a ½ tip (or snip off the corner of a plastic bag).

4. Combine egg whites and lemon juice.

5. Beat with an electric mixture until the whites hold into stiff peaks.

6. Beat xylitol into the mix 1 Tbsp. at a time until fully dissolved. Test a small amount of mixture by rubbing in-between your fingers. You should not be able to feel any granules when the mixture is ready.

7. When the meringue is very stiff and glossy, transfer it into the pastry bag.

8. Hold the bag perpendicular to the baking sheet and pipe 2" high mounds.

9. Bake for 2 hours, then turn the oven off, leaving the meringues in the cooling oven overnight.

10. If the meringues are still sticky then next day, leave

them in the over or another dry place until they are no longer tacky to the touch.

Lemon-Ginger-Kale Smoothie

Servings: 1

Ingredients

¼ cup egg whites
½ cup water
½ cup ice cubes
juice of 1 lemon
fresh ginger, peeled, sliced 1" thick
1 cup kale, packed
pinch of sea salt
stevia to taste

Directions

1. Blend all ingredients together until smooth

Chapter Five

PHASE THREE

PHASE THREE IS all about eating fat to lose weight. That may seem counter-intuitive, but the healthy fats from nuts, olives, and avocados are going to tell your body to burn not just dietary fat, but also stored fat. Your body is ready to do this because you have followed phases one and two and done the prep work.

All week you have kept your fat intake pretty low while flooding your body with vegetables, proteins and whole grains. Because you haven't been eating fats, the body has burned its fat stores for energy. Now, your body is getting suspicious – and this is why so many low-fat, low-carb diets fail. As you first lose weight, the body begins to store fat instead of burning it.

That's why you need to increase your fat intake in the third phase.

Healthy fats do a lot more than just help you lose weight, though. When you eat plenty of healthy fats like those found in avocados, nuts and olive oil, you help satiate your body and relieve stress. And when our stress levels are lower, cortisol hormone levels are lower, too. This helps prevent stress-induced weight gain. In order to enhance the effect in phase three, the emphasis is on stress-reducing exercises such as massage and yoga techniques. These will help you lower your stress levels and promote the release of toxins trapped in the body's cells.

The foods you'll consume in phase three are rich in choline and inositol, elements that metabolize fat and keep it from getting stuck in the liver.

Additionally in phase three, eating fatty fish such as salmon will help promote a healthy hormone balance in the adrenal glands and thyroid. This helps slow gastric emptying and makes you feel full longer. In turn, this stimulates your hypothalamus and pituitary glands, which manufacture the brain release feel-good hormones.

Foods to Eat and Avoid

[Remember to multiply by 1.5 if you need to lose 20 to 40 pounds and by 2 if you need to lose over 40 pounds.]

- *Vegetables* – unlimited
- *Protein* – 4 oz. meat, 6 oz. fish, ½ cup legumes
- *Eggs* – 1 whole
- *Grains* – ½ cup cooked or ½ oz. crackers
- *Fruit* – 1 piece or 1 cup
- *Fat* – ½ avocado, **1/3** cup hummus, ¼ cup raw nuts, 2 tablespoons seed or nut butter, 3 tablespoons of oils, 2-4 tablespoons salad dressing
- *Smoothies* – 1 12oz. glass

Safe Foods

- *Vegetables and Salad Greens*

artichokes, arrowroot, asparagus, arugula, bean sprouts, avocados, beets, beans, bok choy, beet greens, Brussels sprouts, broccoli, cabbage, butternut squash, cauliflower, carrots, chicory, celery, cucumbers, collard greens, endive, eggplant, garlic, fennel, green onions, green chilis, peppers, onions, mixed greens, mushrooms, okra, olives, leeks, kohlrabi, lettuce, rhubarb, radishes, shallots, seaweed, spirulina, spinach, sweet potatoes, tomatoes, winter squash, watercress, zucchini

● *Fruits*
blueberries, blackberries, cherries, cranberries, lemons, grapefruit, limes, plums, peaches, raspberries, prickly pears, rhubarb
coconut milk, coconut, coconut cream, coconut water

● *Animal Protein*
beef, buffalo, lamb, pork, liver, rabbit, chicken, turkey, game, deli meats, corned beef, turkey bacon, sausages, herring, halibut, salmon, sardines, sea bass, trout, skate tuna, clams, calamari, crabs, lobster meat, scallops, oysters, shrimp, whole eggs

● *Vegetable Protein*
beans, chickpeas, black-eyed peas, lentils, almond cheese, almond milk, almond flour, hemp milk, cashew milk, vegan cheddar cheese, nuts and seeds

● *Grains and Starch*
barley, quinoa, oats, sprouted grain, wild rice, black rice, nut flours, brown rice, rice milk, brown rice milk, tapioca, arrowroot, tapioca flour

● *Broth, Herbs, Spices and Condiments*
arrowroot, baking soda, baking powder, broth, Brewer's yeast, Dijon mustard (sugar-free), cream of

tartar, horseradish, dill pickles (sugar-free), mustard, ketchup (no added sugar or corn syrup), natural seasonings, liquid smoke, salsa, raw cocoa powder, tomato sauce, tamari, vanilla extract, tomato paste, vinegar, peppermint extract, balsamic vinegar, apple cider vinegar, coconut vinegar, red wine vinegar, malt vinegar, white vinegar
fresh or dried herbs
spices

● *Sweeteners*
Xylitol

● *Grains and Starch*
barley, amaranth, brown rice, black barley, kamut, buckwheat, spelt, quinoa, sprouted grain, triticale, teff, wild rice
nut flours
brown rice milk, cheese and rice milk
tapioca and arrowroot flour

● *Healthy Fats*
avocados, nuts, olives, coconut milk, coconut cream, almond milk, almond cream, hemp milk, cashew milk, raw seeds, nut butters, coconut oil, olive oil, grapeseed oil, sesame oil, hummus, safflower mayonnaise

● *Beverages*
water

non-caffeinated herbal tea

Unsafe Foods

- Roasted peanuts
- Any food not listed above

Increasing Exercise

This phase is all about allowing your body to relax and heal after the strenuous exercises in phase two. Try to get in two 30-minute sessions of yoga for the three days you're in this phase. You can also try meditation in the morning, and going to get a massage in the afternoon.

Sample Meal Plan

You'll be eating three meals and two snacks every three to four hours each day. Be sure to eat enough healthy fats every day.

- *Breakfast* – have a fruit, fatty protein, grain and veggie within thirty minutes of waking.

- *Snack* – have a vegetable and fatty protein three hours later.
- *Lunch* – have a fatty protein, vegetable and fruit three hours later.
- *Snack* – have a vegetable and fatty protein three hours later.
- *Dinner* – have a fatty protein, vegetable and grain three to four hours later.

You'll be in this phase of the program for three days out of the week, so Friday, Saturday, and Sunday.

Chapter Six

PHASE THREE RECIPES

Easy Breakfast Recipes
Cacao-Crunch Pancakes

Servings: 4

Ingredients

1 cup gluten-free flour
1 Tbsp. Xylitol
½ tsp. salt

3 Tbsp. cacao nibs
2 tsp. baking powder
1 cup almond milk
2 Tbsp. olive oil
1 egg
1 tsp. ground cinnamon
1 tsp. vanilla extract
8 oz. cooked turkey bacon
blueberries or raspberries
1 jicama, peeled and sliced

Directions

1. Combine the milk, oil, egg and vanilla with a mixer. Add the flour, baking powder, Xylitol, cinnamon and salt. Mix until just combined.

2. Heat a skillet and pour the pancakes in. Sprinkle some cacao nibs on each pancake.

3. Cook until bubbles form. Flip and cook another two minutes.
Makes a dozen pancakes.

Blueberry, Avocado, Coconut Smoothie

Serves: 1

Ingredients

¾ cup water
¼ cup coconut kefir
four ice cubes
1 cup spinach
1 cup blueberries
¼ avocado

Directions

1. Place everything in a blender and pulse. Thin it with a little water if the mixture is too thick.

Chicken Avocado BLT Wraps

Serves: 2

Ingredients

* *Vinaigrette*
¼ cup olive oil
1 ½ Tbsp. balsamic vinegar
½ tsp. Dijon mustard
½ tsp. garlic, minced
salt and ground black pepper

* *Wraps*
4 cups mixed salad greens
4 oz. chicken, cooked and shredded
4 oz. turkey bacon, cooked and chopped
1 avocado, sliced
1 cup cherry tomatoes
2 tortilla shells , salt and ground black pepper

Directions

1. Shake the vinaigrette ingredients together in a jar. Toss with greens.

2. Stuff the greens and wrap ingredients into the tortillas and sprinkle with salt and pepper.
To complete each phase three breakfast, serve with a cup of berries, two ounces of bacon and sliced jicama.

Nutty Granola

Serves: 12

Ingredients

3 cups old-fashioned oats
½ cup raisins
1/3 cup walnuts, chopped
1/3 cup raw sunflower seed kernels
¼ cup raw wheat germ
¼ cup flaked unsweetened coconut
¼ cup apple juice
Zest of on orange
1 Tbsp. coconut oil, melted
1 tsp cinnamon
¼ tsp salt

Directions

1. Preheat ovan to 300 degrees F.

2. Spray 10 ½" x 15 ½" pan with nonstick cooking (preferably coconut oil) spray.

3. Combine all ingredients (expect raisins) and mix

well.

4. Spread mixture evenly onto prepared pan.

5. Bake for 25 minutes, stirring once, until lightly browned.

6. Let mixture cool.

7. Mix raisins into cooled mixture.

8. Can be stored in covered container and used as needed.

Quick Lunch Recipes
Chicken and Roasted Red Pepper Frittata

Servings: 4

Ingredients

half onion, sliced
6 egg whites
8 oz. skinless, boneless, cooked chicken breast
½ cup jarred roasted red peppers
½ tsp. Italian seasoning

¼ tsp. salt

4 basil leaves

Directions

1. Preheat the oven to 325 degrees F.

2. In a skillet, sauté the onion for about seven minutes.

3. In another bowl, whip the egg whites until they're frothy, around 30 seconds.

4. When the onions are done, stir in the chicken, seasoning, peppers and salt. Then pour the mixture into a baking pan containing the egg whites.

5. Sprinkle basil over the top. Place the pan in the oven and bake for ten minutes.

6. Slide the frittata out of the pan and onto a cutting board and slice into four wedges.

Three-Minute Asparagus-Shrimp Stir Fry

Serves: 4

Ingredients

1 lb. shrimp, prepared
2 Tbsp. grapeseed oil
1 lb. asparagus, trimmed
1 Tbsp. garlic, minced
1 Tbsp. ginger, grated
¼ tsp. crushed red pepper flakes
2 Tbsp. tamari
2 tsp. sesame oil
2 cups cooked quinoa

Directions

1. Heat a skillet over high heat and add oil. Stir-fry the shrimp for one minute or until they're pink. Remove to a plate and leave the oil in the pan.

2. Add the asparagus, stir-frying for one minute. Add the ginger, garlic and red pepper flakes and stir. Return the shrimp to the pan and stir-fry another minute.

3. Remove and place everything into a bowl. Toss it with the tamari and oil, and then serve it over the quinoa.

Mix-and-Match Kebabs

Servings: 4

Ingredients

lamb, chicken breast or beef filet cut in 1" cubes (6 oz. for each kebab)

¼ cup water

1 cup balsamic vinegar

3 Tbsp. Dijon mustard

¼ cup lemon juice

2 tsp. garlic, minced

1 tsp. parsley flakes

¼ tsp. ground black pepper

¼ tsp. salt

1 packet Xylitol

fennel chunks

peach quarters

Directions

1. Alternate meat, vegetables and fruit on the skewers. Place them into a shallow container and marinate with remaining ingredients for two hours.

1. Bake or grill for ten minutes, turning the kebabs once.

Chicken Chili

Servings: 6

Ingredients

4-5 chicken breasts, cubed
6 scallions, chopped
1 bell pepper, diced
4 ribs of celery, finely diced
1 clove garlic, chopped
1 10 oz. can Rotel® died tomatoes with chiles
5 Tbsp. olive oil
2 tsp. butter
2 cups chicken stock
¾ cup water
1 tbsp. chili powder (or more depending on your spice comfort)
1 tsp. cumin
Salt and pepper to taste
grated parmesan cheese for garnish

Directions

1. In a hot skillet, sauté scallions, celery and bell pepper in butter.

2. Add chicken and cook just until the color begins to turn brown.

3. In a crockpot set to warm, combine chicken stock, canned tomatoes, water, garlic, cumin and chili powder.

4. Add the chicken and vegetables into the crockpot. Stir to blend.

5. Cover and cook on high for one hour.

6. Turn heat to low and cook for another 4-5 hours.

7. Serve in a bowl and garnish with parmesan cheese.

Simple Dinner Recipes

Garden Meatballs

Servings: 6

Ingredients

½ lb. ground turkey
1 lb. ground beef

4 cups spinach, chopped
½ cup celery, chopped
4 scallions, chopped
1 bell pepper, chopped
1/3 cup chili paste
2 Tbsp. tamari
7 oz. mild green chilis, diced
1 tsp. salt
½ tsp. ground black pepper

Directions

1. Preheat your oven to 375 degrees F.

2. In a bowl, combine the ingredients. With damp palms, roll the meat mixture into balls and place them in a 9"x13" baking dish.

3. Bake for 35 minutes, turning the meatballs every 15 minutes.

4. Serve warm or refrigerate for later.

Shrimp with Spinach Fettuccine

Servings: 2

Ingredients

2 packets spinach fettuccine
12 oz. shrimp, prepared
¾ tsp. salt
½ tsp. red pepper flakes
4 Tbsp. olive oil
1 onion, sliced
14 ½ oz. diced tomatoes
3 cloves garlic, chopped
¼ tsp. oregano
3 Tbsp. Italian parsley, chopped
3 Tbsp. basil leaves chopped

Directions

1. Prepare the noodles according to instructions and set aside in a bowl.

2. Toss the shrimp with the red pepper flakes and salt. Heat the oil in a skillet and sauté the shrimp for two minutes or until they're pink. Remove the shrimp and set aside. Add the onion to the skillet and sauté five

minutes. Add the tomatoes, oregano, and garlic and sauté another two minutes.

3. Return the shrimp and juices to the mix and toss to coat. Cook another minute and stir in the basil and parsley.

4. Season with salt and serve over the noodles.

Classic Maryland Crab Cakes

Servings: 4

Ingredients

18 oz. lump grade crabmeat
1 egg
¼ cup safflower mayonnaise
1 ½ tsp. Dijon mustard
1 ½ tsp. Old Bay® seasoning
1 tsp. lemon juice
salt
1 ¼ cup breadcrumbs
1 Tbsp. flat leaf parsley, chopped
3 Tbsp. olive oil
lemon wedges

Directions

1. Drain the meat and remove shell pieces. Put in a mixing bowl and set aside.

2. In a bowl, whisk the mayonnaise, egg, mustard, lemon juice, seasoning and a quarter teaspoon of salt together. Mix with crab until well combined.

3. Break up any lumps with your fingers.

4. Sprinkle the mixture with the crumbs and parsley. Mix thoroughly and gently. You want the mix to be loose and not turn to mush. Cover and refrigerate one to three hours.

5. Shape the mix into eight patties about an inch thick. In a skillet, heat oil and add the cakes. Cook until they're dark golden brown on the bottom, around four minutes. Reduce the heat to low and cook another four to five minutes on the other side.

6. Serve with lemon wedges.

Thai Basil Ground Turkey and Eggplant

Servings: 4

Ingredients

1 lb ground turkey or chicken
1-2 eggplants cut into irregular shapes
4-8 cabbage or lettuce leaves
½ green pepper, sliced
½ red pepper, sliced
½ red onion, sliced
2 carrots, julienned
1 cup fresh basil leaves
1 cup chicken broth
2 Tbsp. extra-virgin olive oil
2 Tbsp. minced garlic
2 Tbsp. soy sauce
1 package Stevia sweetener (equivalent to 2 tsp sugar)
juice from ½ lime
1-2 jalapeño peppers, chopped (optional)

Directions

1. Heat oil in wok or skillet.

2. Add garlic and sauté until lightly browned.

3. Mix in onion and ground turkey or chicken until meat is cooked.

4. Add sliced peppers, julienned carrots, eggplant chunks, basil leaves, chopped jalapeño, soy sauce, Stevia, lime juice, and chicken broth.

5. Cook until vegetables are soft but not mushy, or until basil has wilted.

6. Serve over a bed of cabbage or lettuce leaves.

Zucchini Fries

Servings: 3

Ingredients

2 zucchini
2 egg whites
1 cup breadcrumbs
1 tsp. salt
¼ tsp. garlic powder
¼ tsp. ground black pepper

Directions

1. Pat and clean the zucchini, and cut it into ½" thick

wedges.

2. Beat the egg whites in a bowl. Mix the crumbs with the seasonings on a plate.

3. Dip the zucchini into the egg white, allow excess to drip off, and then roll it in the breadcrumbs and seasoning.

4. Spread zucchini pieces onto a greased baking sheet and bake at 450 degrees F for ten minutes on each side.

Cheesy Jalapeno Mini Cornbread Muffins

Servings: 12

Ingredients

¾ cup whole wheat flour (or brown rice flour, or rye flour)
¾ cup ground cornmeal
½ cup (2 oz.) shredded reduced-fat cheddar cheese
2 egg whites
1 jalapeño pepper, minced
¾ cup nonfat milk

3 Tbsp. extra-virgin olive oil

2 Tbsp. agave nectar

1 tsp. baking powder

¼ tsp. baking soda

¼ tsp. smoked paprika

¼ tsp. cumin

¼ tsp. salt

Directions

1. Preheat oven to 400 degrees F.

2. Spray 24-mini-muffin cups with nonstick coconut oil cooking spray.

3. Combine cheese and jalapeño in a small bowl and set aside.

4. Combine flour, cornmeal, baking powder, baking soda, cumin, paprika, and salt into a large bowl and mix well.

5. Whisk milk egg whites, oil, and agave in a medium bowl until smooth and blended well.

6. Stir wet mixture into flour mixture until fully combined.

7. Spoon 1 tsp batter into each mini-muffin cup.

8. Place ½ tsp cheese mixture into center of each mini-muffin cup.

9. Add another 1 tsp batter to each mini-muffin cup covering the cheese.

10. Bake 10 minutes or until lightly golden brown.

11. Cool in the pan on a wire rack for at least 5 minutes.

12. Remove from pan to wire rack.

13. Serve warm or cool.

Walnut Sunflower Bread

Servings: 4

Ingredients

2/3 cup rye flour
1/3 cup spelt flour

2-3 Tbsp. Dry active yeast

2 Tbsp. extra-virgin coconut oil

1 Tbsp. salt

2 Tbsp. ground flaxseed

3 Tbsp. sunflower seeds

1 handful walnuts, chopped

160 ml warm water

ground coriander, aniseed, and cardamom to taste

[It is possible to use different flour types and oils for this recipe to create different breads.]

Directions

1. Preheat oven to 500 degrees F.

2. In a large bowl, mix all ingredients.

3. Knead dough for about 5 minutes, until all the flour is worked into the dough (you can do this by hand or use a handheld mixer)

4. Cover and let rice is a warm place for 45 minutes.

5. Punch down the dough and work it on a floured board for another 5 minutes, until it is not sticky anymore.

6. Place back in bowl, cover it, and let rise another 30 minutes.

7. Punch down again. Form a loaf shape and either put into a small loaf pan or place onto parchment-covered baking tray.

8. Place in oven and reduce temperature to 475 degrees F.

9. Place a small pan with water in the bottom of the oven to keep the loaf moist.

10. Bake for 15 minutes.

11. Reduce temperature to 400 degrees F. and bake for another 30 minutes.

Creamy Ranch Dressing

Servings: 2-4 Tbsp. is a serving

Ingredients

- *Spice Mix*
¼ cup parsley

2 tsp. dill
2 tsp. onion powder
1 ½ tsp. basil
1 ½ tsp. salt
1 tsp. ground black pepper
½ tsp. garlic powder

● *Dressing*
2/3 cup safflower mayonnaise
3 Tbsp. almond milk
¼ tsp. vinegar

Directions

1. Mix together dry spice mix ingredients in a jar.

2. Stir in remaining ingredients until thoroughly combined.

3. Store in a jar in the refrigerator.

Snacks and Desserts
Carrot-Oat Breakfast Cookies

Servings: 6

Ingredients

1 cup rolled oats

¾ cup Bob's Red Mill® biscuit and baking mix

1 ½ tsp. baking powder

1 ½ tsp. cinnamon

½ cup Xylitol

1 egg

¾ cup grated carrot

¼ cup almond milk

1 Tbsp. coconut oil

¾ cup walnuts, chopped

Directions

1. Preheat your oven to 375 degrees F.

2. Whisk the dry ingredients together. In another bowl, beat the egg, carrot, oil and milk. Add the wet ingredients to the dry and stir to combine. Fold in the nuts. Drop twelve cookies onto a parchment paper-lined baking sheet.

3. Bake 12 to 15 minutes or until the bottoms are lightly browned.

Crockpot Berry Bread Pudding

Serves: 12 servings

Ingredients

6 cups bread, cut into 1" cubes
½ cup toasted almonds, slivered
6 large eggs, beaten
1 ¾ cup low-fat milk
1 ½ tsp. ground cinnamon
1 tsp. vanilla
dark agave (equivalent to 1 ½ cups brown sugar)
3 cups strawberries, sliced
2 cups blueberries
1 cup raisins

Directions

1. Coat crockpot with nonstick spray.

2. Combine bread, almonds, and raisins into crockpot.

3. Whisk together milk, eggs, agave and cinnamon into a separate bowl.

4. Pour mixture over bread and gently combine all

ingredients.

5. Cover and heat on low for 4 hours

6. Remove center pot from heating element and allow bread pudding to cool before serving. Pudding will firm as it cools.

7. Serve with berries over the top.

Vanilla Cake Bites

Serves: 12 servings

Ingredients

4 egg whites
½ cup unsweetened almond milk
3 Tbsp. unsweetened applesauce
1 tsp vanilla extract
1 cup whole wheat flour
2 scoops vanilla protein powder
1 oz. sugar-free vanilla pudding mix
6 tsp. stevia blend
¼ tsp baking powder

Directions

1. Preheat oven to 350 degrees F.

2. Combine all dry ingredients until fully mixed together.

3. Combine all wet ingredients.

4. Slowly mix dry ingredients into wet ingredients, stirring until no dry ingredients can be seen.

5. Pour batter into mini-bite or small muffin pans

6. Bake for 9 minutes, checking to ensure a wooden toothpick can be inserted and withdrawn without any batter sticking to the toothpick.

Spicy Ranchero Deviled Eggs, Peppers & Tomatoes

Serves: 6-8 servings

Ingredients

8 hard boiled eggs, pealed & halved on long side

4 Roma tomatoes

4 jalapeños

½ cup plain Greek yogurt

¼ cup thinly sliced green onions

3 Tbsp. + 1 tsp. extra-virgin olive oil

2 Tbs. cilantro

1 oz creamy ranch dressing dry spice mix

● *Creamy Ranch Dressing Spice Mix*

¼ cup parsley

2 tsp. dill

2 tsp. onion powder

1 ½ tsp. basil

1 ½ tsp. salt

1 tsp. ground black pepper

½ tsp. garlic powder

Directions

1. Coat a skillet with 1 tsp. olive oil and place over medium heat.

2. Add whole peppers to hot skillet and cook for about 5 minutes or until lightly charred. Turn occasionally.

3. Let peppers cool.

4. Halve peppers, removing seeds and membranes.

5. Scoop out tomato halves and set aside.

6. Remove yolks from eggs and place in a bowl.

7. Add 4 of the egg white halves to the bowl and mash together.

8. Stir in yogurt, green onions, cilantro, dressing powder, and the remainder of the olive oil. Mix together well.

9. Spoon mixture into the egg white halves, Chili peppers tomatoes.'

10. Chill in the refrigerator until 20 minutes before serving.

You now have a clear idea of what you're able to eat for all three phases, so let's take a look at the full 28-day plan to get you started on the Carb Cycling Diet!

Chapter Seven

FULL 28 DAY PLAN

THE CARB CYCLING Diet requires that you switch what you're eating every few days. For the first two days, you'll be following phase one of the diet. The second two days will be the second phase of the diet, and the last three days will be the third phase of the diet. You will be using three different types of exercises during the week, so you should never get bored with what you're eating or doing!

However, you do have to have a strategy in order to successfully complete this diet. That's because it's unlike any other diet out there. This diet requires that you eat something from every food group, but not in the same day. It's not about counting calories, so you thankfully don't have to worry about that. But it is about eating the proper foods at the right times in order to get your metabolism back in shape. Think of your metabolism like a muscle – you want to strengthen it, so you have to work it out a bit to get it to be stronger.

Phases

As a refresher, let's go over how much you're going to eat in each phase one more time. Then I'll outline your plan for you.

Phase One – The Adrenals

Remember that this phase is about giving your adrenal system a break. In the first phase, you'll need to eat three meals with high amounts of healthy carbohydrates, a moderate amount of protein and a low amount of fat. This will soothe the adrenals and make you feel less stressed.

You'll also be performing cardiovascular workouts in

the first phase to help clean out the adrenals and restore cortisol hormone levels that are appropriate to your body.

Phase Two – Rebuilding Muscle

The second phase of the diet is about rebuilding your muscles by consuming low amounts of fat, low amounts of carbohydrates, and high amounts of protein. Protein is the building block for muscles, and for other organs in your body that are also made of muscle. Muscle continues to burn calories even while you're sedentary, so it's a good thing to have if you want to reach and remain at your goal weight.

In this phase, you'll need to perform muscle focused exercises, such as lifting free weights or using your body weight as resistance against gravity. If you're overweight and have less than ideal muscle mass, then you want to begin with lifting only your own body weight. You can move on to small free weights after you've dropped a few pounds.

Phase Three – Eating Fat to Lose Fat

The third phase of the diet is about eating more fat, in order to lose fat. By the time you reach this phase, the body has been programmed to use fat as a fuel source. Yet you don't want to lose too much of it too quickly. If you quit after phase two and don't continue with this part of the program, your body may rebel and stop burning fat as fuel. To keep the body happily burning fat, you have to supplement that fat supply.

In the third phase, you'll be doing a lot of relaxing exercises in order to stay stress-free. This phase is all about activities such as getting massage therapy to help the body heal or taking yoga classes in order to keep it limber while it does so.

Meal Plan

So you've heard enough of an overview of the phases! Let's explore the 28-day plan that will help you lose weight healthily and quickly!

Week One Meal Plan

	Breakfast	**Morning Snack**	**Lunch**	**Afternoon Snack**	**Dinner**
Week One Phase 1					
Day 1	Egg White Soufflé with dry toast	Tex-Mex Black Bean Dip with sliced vegetables	Easy Oven Fajitas and fruit side	Orange Slices	Slow Cooker Balsamic Turkey Roast and Roasted Cabbage with Mustard Vinaigrette
Day 2	Non-fat Yogurt with Fruit	Chocolate Drizzled Stuffed Strawberries	DIY Pizza and fruit side	Tex-Mex Black Bean Dip with sliced vegetables	Jambalaya and Garden Salad with Italian Dressing
Week One Phase 2					
Day 3	Homemade Breakfast Sausage with egg whites	Power Protein Dip with sliced vegetables	Chicken, Red Pepper and Basil Lettuce Wrap	Lemon-Ginger-Kale Smoothie	Lettuce Wraps with Smoked Salmon and Cauliflower Fried Rice
Day 4	Sweet Potato and Squash Pancakes	Lemon Meringue Puffs	Salad Nicoise	Power Protein Dip with sliced vegetables	Glazed Pork Tenderloin with Horseradish Sauce and Sautéed Leeks
Week One Phase 3					
Day 5	Blueberry, Avocado, Coconut Smoothie	Carrot-Oat Breakfast Cookies	Chicken and Roasted Red Pepper Frittata	Crockpot Berry Bread Pudding	Garden Meatballs and Zucchini Fries
Day 6	Chicken Avocado BLT Wraps	Crockpot Berry Bread Pudding	Three-Minute Asparagus-Shrimp Stir Fry	Vanilla Cake Bites	Shrimp with Spinach Fettuccine and Garden Salad with Creamy Ranch Dressing
Day 7	Cacao-Crunch Pancakes	Spicy Ranchero Deviled Eggs, Peppers & Tomatoes	Mix-and-Match Kebabs	Carrot-Oat Breakfast Cookies	Classic Maryland Crab Cakes and Cheesy Jalapeno Mini Cornbread Muffins

Week Two Meal Plan

	Breakfast	Morning Snack	Lunch	Afternoon Snack	Dinner
Week Two Phase 1					
Day 1	Veggie Frittata	Orange Slices	Grilled Chicken & Apple Salad (with Apple Cider Vinaigrette Dressing)	Chocolate Drizzled Stuffed Strawberries	Lemon Chicken with Feta and Green Beans with Shallots and Mushrooms
Day 2	Non-fat Yogurt with Fruit	Tex-Mex Black Bean Dip with sliced vegetables	Easy Oven Fajitas and fruit side	Orange Slices	Slow Cooker Balsamic Turkey Roast and Roasted Cabbage with Mustard Vinaigrette
Week Two Phase 2					
Day 3	Fat-Blasting Baked Egg Casserole	Lemon-Ginger-Kale Smoothie	Chicken, Red Pepper and Basil Lettuce Wrap	Lemon Meringue Puffs	Baked Fish with Lemons and Creamy Broccoli & Carrots Stir-fry
Day 4	Homemade Breakfast Sausage with egg whites	Power Protein Dip with sliced vegetables	Sweet Potato Soup	Lemon-Ginger-Kale Smoothie	Lettuce Wraps with Smoked Salmon and Cauliflower Fried Rice
Week Two Phase 3					
Day 5	Nutty Granola	Vanilla Cake Bites	Chicken Chili	Spicy Ranchero Deviled Eggs, Peppers & Tomatoes	Thai Basil Ground Turkey and Eggplant and Walnut Sunflower Bread
Day 6	Blueberry, Avocado, Coconut Smoothie	Spicy Ranchero Deviled Eggs, Peppers & Tomatoes	Chicken and Roasted Red Pepper Frittata	Carrot-Oat Breakfast Cookies	Garden Meatballs and Zucchini Fries
Day 7	Cacao-Crunch Pancakes	Carrot-Oat Breakfast Cookies	Three-Minute Asparagus-Shrimp Stir Fry	Vanilla Cake Bites	Shrimp with Spinach Fettuccine and Garden Salad with Creamy Ranch Dressing

Week Three Meal Plan

CTL - Carb	Breakfast	Morning Snack	Lunch	Afternoon Snack	Dinner
Week Three Phase 1					
Day 1	Non-fat Yogurt with Fruit	Chocolate Drizzled Stuffed Strawberries	DIY Pizza and fruit side	Orange Slices	Jambalaya and Garden Salad with Italian Dressing
Day 2	Egg-White Soufflé with dry toast	Orange Slices	Grilled Chicken & Apple Salad (with Apple Cider Vinaigrette Dressing)	Tex-Mex Black Bean Dip with sliced vegetables	Lemon Chicken with Feta and Green Beans with Shallots and Mushrooms
Week Three Phase 2					
Day 3	Sweet Potato and Squash Pancakes	Protein Dip with sliced vegetables	Salad Nicoise	Lemon-Ginger-Kale Smoothie	Glazed Pork Tenderloin with Horseradish Sauce and Sautéed Leeks
Day 4	Fat-Blasting Baked Egg Casserole	Lemon-Ginger-Kale Smoothie	Sweet Potato Soup	Lemon Meringue Puffs	Baked Fish with Lemons and Creamy Broccoli & Carrots Stir-fry
Week Three Phase 3					
Day 5	Cacao-Crunch Pancakes	Spicy Ranchero Deviled Eggs, Peppers & Tomatoes	Mix-and-Match Kebabs	Crockpot Berry Bread Pudding	Shrimp with Spinach Fettuccine and Garden Salad with Creamy Ranch Dressing
Day 6	Blueberry, Avocado, Coconut Smoothie	Vanilla Cake Bites	Chicken Chili	Spicy Ranchero Deviled Eggs, Peppers & Tomatoes	Classic Maryland Crab Cakes and Cheesy Jalapeno Mini Cornbread Muffins
Day 7	Chicken Avocado BLT Wraps	Crockpot Berry Bread Pudding	Three-Minute Asparagus-Shrimp Stir Fry	Carrot-Oat Breakfast Cookies	Thai Basil Ground Turkey and Eggplant and Walnut Sunflower Bread

Week Four Meal Plan

	Breakfast	**Morning Snack**	**Lunch**	**Afternoon Snack**	**Dinner**
Week Four Phase 1					
Day 1	Veggie Frittata	Orange Slices	Easy Oven Fajitas and fruit side	Orange Slices	Lemon Chicken with Feta and Green Beans with Shallots and Mushrooms
Day 2	Egg-White Soufflé with dry toast	Tex-Mex Black Bean Dip with sliced vegetables	Grilled Chicken & Apple Salad (with Apple Cider Vinaigrette Dressing)	Chocolate Drizzled Stuffed Strawberries	Slow Cooker Balsamic Turkey Roast and Roasted Cabbage with Mustard Vinaigrette
Week Four Phase 2					
Day 3	Homemade Breakfast Sausage with egg whites	Lemon Meringue Puffs	Sweet Potato Soup	Lemon Meringue Puffs	Baked Fish with Lemons and Creamy Broccoli & Carrots Stir-fry
Day 4	Fat-Blasting Baked Egg Casserole	Lemon-Ginger-Kale Smoothie	Chicken, Red Pepper and Basil Lettuce Wrap	Protein Dip with sliced vegetables	Glazed Pork Tenderloin with Horseradish Sauce and Sautéed Leeks
Week Four Phase 3					
Day 5	Chicken Avocado BLT Wraps	Crockpot Berry Bread Pudding	Three-Minute Asparagus-Shrimp Stir Fry	Vanilla Cake Bites	Classic Maryland Crab Cakes and Cheesy Jalapeno Mini Cornbread Muffins
Day 6	Nutty Granola	Vanilla Cake Bites	Mix-and-Match Kebabs	Carrot-Oat Breakfast Cookies	Garden Meatballs and Zucchini Fries
Day 7	Blueberry, Avocado, Coconut Smoothie	Carrot-Oat Breakfast Cookies	Chicken and Roasted Red Pepper Frittata	Crockpot Berry Bread Pudding	Shrimp with Spinach Fettuccine and Garden Salad with Creamy Ranch Dressing

That's your 28-day meal plan! Keep in mind that you can substitute any other recipes you find that will fit the requirements for each phase. For example, if you're a busy person and don't have time to make lunch, then you can substitute a salad with chicken on top during phase two. Just be sure you're getting the right amount of vegetables, protein and carbohydrates in each phase.

A common problem people have is that vegetables, fruits and dips go bad before they're able to use them the next week. Don't be afraid to experiment with frozen fruits and vegetables! That way you can use whatever you need and freeze the rest. Keep in mind that you can also freeze leftovers for the following day or the following week. That way you're not wasting food.

Now that you know how to plan out your first week, let's talk about exercising.

Exercise Plan

Each phase is going to emphasize a different type of exercise. But they are all very simple to do and you only have to exercise once during phase one and phase two! You should probably try to do all three of the phase three activities each week.

Exercise Activity

All Weeks Phase 1

Day 1	Cardio for 15 minutes (walking briskly, jogging, Stair Climbing, Calisthenics, etc.)
Day 2	Take a Break

All Weeks Phase 2

Day 3	Body Building: 8 Lunges 6 Bicep Curls 4 Push-Ups
Day 4	Take a Break

All Weeks Phase 3

Day 5	Get a Message
Day 6	Take a 1 Hour Yoga Class
Day 7	Meditate for 30 Minutes

For weeks two, three and four you can repeat these exercises. If you feel comfortable by week four, you can add some hand-weights to your lunges and bicep curls to make them more effective. Remember to only exercise once during the first two phases! If you overdo it, the body will rebel and you'll be left weighing more than when you started!

CONCLUSION

The 28-day plan that has been laid out for you is not complex. In fact, it should be fairly easy for you to follow and complete. That is the good news. But this plan will not work by itself. It is up to you to take action. Don't put down this book and go right back to your old routine. Instead, make the decision to start changing your life so that you can achieve your goal.

1. Create a shopping list of foods that you will need for the current week's menu. For extra credit, you can create a shopping list for all four weeks of the plan so that you will be prepared and have no excuses until it comes time to buy groceries again.

2. Set aside a specific time in your calendar to follow the exercise plan. You don't want to allow for any excuses for not doing your scheduled activities. Remember to start slow and work your way up to more vigorous activities.

3. Make sure you include time in each day to unwind and relax. Many people find joining a yoga class helps. But I am sure you can find plenty of alternatives, even if it is just getting some quiet time to yourself to read a good book.

4. Seek out a partner or group of friends who also want to lose weight and get into better physical shape. It always helps to be surrounded by friends who can support you. This is the very best way to ensure that you do continue with your plan. When you feel like quitting or "cheating" on the diet, your partner will be there to offer you encouragement. And when they experience a moment of weakness, you will be there to motivate them to continue.

5. Stay positive. Look forward to a better tomorrow. If you don't have hope, you will become discouraged. If you can imagine a better tomorrow, you will be encouraged to keep your newfound habits and begin to live a happy life again.

Thank you for purchasing this book! I hope it has helped you in achieving your goals!

BONUS: FREE BOOK PREVIEW:

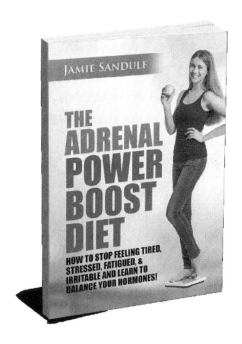

The Adrenal Reset Power Boost Diet
How to Stop Feeling Tired, Stressed, Fatigued &
Irritable and Learn to Balance Your Hormones!

Chapter 1

**What are the true reasons you have these
symptoms?**

Sometimes annoying and unexplainable symptoms haunt us. We may feel weird body aches, unable to concentrate, moodiness or irritability, feel very tired, experience racing thoughts or unexpected cravings for sweet or salty foods. These symptoms may not be bad enough to send us to the doctor, or we may even dismiss them as the effects of aging or just being tired – but when they start to affect our everyday activities and become chronic symptoms, then there may be cause for alarm.

According to Dr. James Wilson, author of the book *"Adrenal Fatigue: The 21ˢᵗ Century Stress Syndrome,"* people may not know that malfunctioning adrenal glands can be the culprit for these unexpected symptoms (along with others that are related to adrenal fatigue). Dr. Wilson has stated that for most people, adrenal fatigue can be relieved with the proper care. If you are suffering from any of the aforementioned symptoms, you can expect to feel better if you get support for your condition, promote healthy adrenal function and, most of all, reduce your stress.

The truth about adrenal fatigue

If you research adrenal fatigue, you will notice that

most of the information you find is either unsupported or contradicts the theory that adrenal fatigue may be the reason behind a variety of health conditions.

People who have sought their doctor's advice for adrenal fatigue have been told that it is not an acknowledged medical condition. There are no drugs to cure adrenal fatigue and, therefore, it is not considered to be part of a conventional medical model. But what people fail to understand is that these nagging symptoms are the body's way of signaling that there is an imbalance. Some ignore the signs or dismiss them and go on with their everyday life. However, for some the symptoms may be very hard to totally overlook.

Prolonged sleeplessness can lead to insomnia and may affect your work, career and your personal relationships. Feeling fatigued and having poor concentration can lead to poor judgment and lack of energy at work and in school. When you ignore adrenal fatigue symptoms, everything important in your life eventually becomes affected.

You need a power boost!

If you are tired of being tired, weak from feeling weak for a long time, then this is the best time to start reviving your life. You can regain your energy and enjoy many of the following benefits when you adopt a Reset Power Boost Diet that is especially designed for people suffering from adrenal fatigue:

- Say goodbye to annoying body aches and start moving again
- Improve your concentration and have a sharper memory
- Improve your mood allowing you to enjoy your life better
- Improve your energy levels
- Correct hormonal imbalances
- Reduce cravings and improve your appetite

The Adrenal Reset Power Boost Diet is a totally new dietary approach to correcting adrenal fatigue. This book will guide you on how this kind of diet can help you regain normal adrenal function and will provide you with amazing energy to power up your day.

There is hope for adrenal fatigue! Let's start making a change now!

Search for "*The Adrenal Reset Power Boost Diet*" on Amazon.com or go to: http://amzn.to/1KEO6Av

OTHER BOOKS BY DIPUGGO PUBLISHING

Below you'll find a list of some of other books from DiPuggo Publishing that are popular on Amazon and Kindle. Simply click on the links below to check them out. Alternatively, visit each author's page on Amazon by clicking on their name below to browse their other works.

Books by Jamie Sandulf:

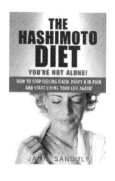

The Hashimoto Diet: You're Not Alone! How to Stop Feeling Tired, Puffy & in Pain … and Start Living Your Life Again!

Often times your doctor and family may make you feel like it is all in your head; that there is nothing wrong with you. But you know that there is something wrong? You're NOT ALONE! Many like you are suffering from this autoimmune disease! And there is hope for you!

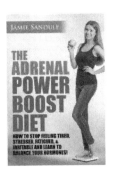

The Adrenal Reset Power Boost Diet: How to Stop Feeling Tired, Stressed, Fatigued & Irritable and Learn to Balance Your Hormones!

Feel More Energetic, Healthy, and Happy on the Adrenal Reset Power Boost Diet!

"The Adrenal Reset Power Boost Diet by Jamie Sandulf approaches the issue from an academic angle. Jamie gives a very illuminating description of the physiological background, the symptoms, as well as the diagnosis of adrenal fatigue. Popular treatments like stress management, yoga, meditation etc. are then discussed, following it with the main theme of this book, a recommended diet plan for promoting adrenal health. Lists indicating popularly available super foods that you can eat today as well as the calories intake are provided, and this enables one to plan appropriate menus. This is a well written book; it answered all the questions that I could pose in this connection. A few references for further study would have been a helpful addition." - ReadersFavorite.com

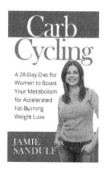

Carb Cycling: A 28-Day Diet for Women to Boost Your Metabolism for Accelerated Fat-Burning Weight Loss

Each year your body's metabolism rate adjusts with your age. By the time you hit 30, you will be losing 1% of your muscle mass every year. So what can you do about it? Crash dieting courses do not work. And hard, intense workouts will not provide the results you are hoping to achieve. Does that make you frustrated? It sure did for me!

The solution is simple. It is right under our noses but we just don't see it. Why? Because we have been blinded by a bombardment of advertising pushing the wrong information at us over and over.

But there is hope! Carb Cycling: A 28-Day Diet for Women makes it simple! Carb cycling is the right way for you to maintain your weight. In this book, you'll find all the necessary elements for achieving a healthy life.

Inspired by real lives, the author tells you why so many women struggle with weight gain. You'll see why this carb cycling diet is easy and the most effective tool for your weight loss. As a bonus, you'll also get a sample diet plan and exercise program.

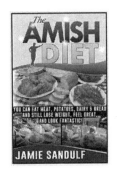

The Amish Diet: You Can Eat Meat, Potatoes, Dairy & Bread and still Lose Weight, Feel Great, and Look Fantastic!

The Amish eat a hearty diet that includes potatoes and meat, yet their communities are not part of the obesity epidemic. Diabetes is rare, and the Amish are significantly healthier than most of the rest of us? What's their secret?

Living With An Alcoholic: How To Take Back Control Of Your Relationship and Save The Person You Love (Alcoholism and Substance Abuse)

You might be wondering how you can best support your loved one as they become sober and battle the illness of alcoholism. This book will provide you with some of the best tools and advice to serve you, your relationship and your well-being throughout this tough situation.

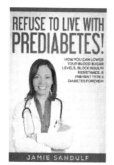

Refuse to Live with Prediabetes! How You Can Lower Your Blood Sugar Levels, Block Insulin Resistance, & Prevent Type II Diabetes Forever!

Once you've been diagnosed with prediabetes your health clock is ticking. For every year after being diagnosed, 10 to 15 percent of patients develop the full-blown disease. That means if you do nothing at all, you will have diabetes within eight to ten year (but probably sooner)!

How to Live Longer: Learn the Secrets of Ancient Cultures on How to Live a Longer, Healthier Life (Anti-Aging Secrets & Home Remedies)

Some ancient civilizations lived to be much older than we do now in most Western cultures. And the people that still live in those areas today have continued to use their secrets to promote very long and satisfying lives.

COMING SOON:

Ketogenic Diet: Guide to Quickly Losing Up to 30 Pounds in 30 Days!.

29242953R00074

Printed in Great Britain
by Amazon